# Lean and Green Diet for Everyone

Improve your Health

and Eat Better

Carmen Bellisario

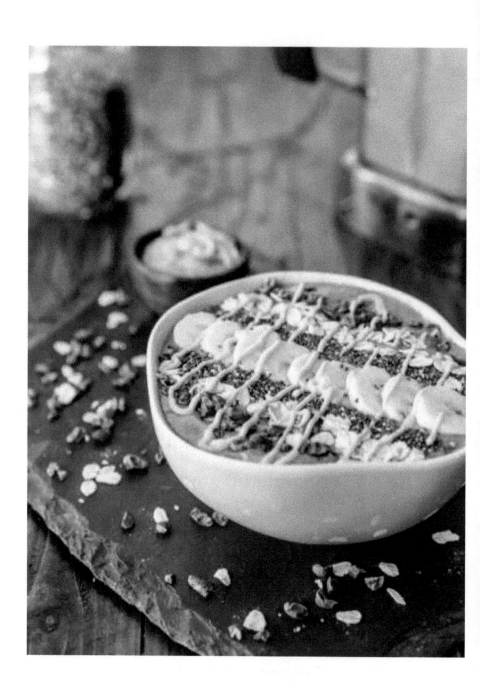

TABLE OF CONTENTS

# Mouth-watering Pie

Preparation time: 15 minutes

Cooking time: 45 minutes

Servings: 8

## Ingredients:

- 3/4-pound of beef; ground
- 1/2 onion; chopped.
- 1 pie crust
- 3 tablespoons of taco seasoning
- 1 teaspoon of baking soda
- Mango salsa for serving
- 1/2 red bell pepper; chopped.
- A handful cilantro; chopped.
- 8 eggs
- 1 teaspoon of coconut oil
- Salt and black pepper to the taste.

## Directions:

1. Heat up a pan, add oil, beef, cook until it browns and mix with salt, pepper, and taco seasoning.

2. Stir again, transfer to a bowl and leave aside for now.

3. Heat up the pan again over medium heat with cooking juices from the meat, add onion and pepper; stir and cook for 4 minutes

4. Add eggs, baking soda and a few salt and stir well.

5. Add cilantro; stir again and start heating.

6. Spread beef mix in pie shell, add veggies mix and cover meat, heat oven at 3500 F and bake for 45 minutes.

7. Leave the pie to chill down a bit, slice, divide between plates and serve with mango salsa on top.

## Nutrition:

- Calories: 198
- Fat: 11 g
- Fiber: 1 g
- Carbs: 12 g
- Protein: 12 g

# Peanut Butter and Cacao Breakfast Quinoa

Preparation time: 5 Minutes

Cooking time: 10 Minutes

Servings: 1

## Ingredients:

- 1/3 cup of quinoa flakes
- 1/2 cup of unsweetened nondairy milk,
- 1/2 cup of water
- 1/8 cup of raw cacao powder
- One tablespoon of natural creamy peanut butter
- 1/8 teaspoon of ground cinnamon
- One banana; mashed
- Fresh berries of choice; for serving
- Chopped nuts of choice; for serving

**Directions:**

1. Using an 8-quart pot over medium-high heat, mix together the quinoa flakes, milk, water, cacao powder, spread, and cinnamon.
2. Cook and stir it until the mixture begins to simmer. Turn the heat to medium-low and cook for 3-5 minutes, stirring frequently.
3. Stir in the bananas and cook until hot.
4. Serve topped with fresh berries, nuts, and a splash of milk.

**Nutrition:**

- Calories: 471
- Fat: 16 g
- Protein: 18 g
- Carbohydrates: 69 g
- Fiber: 16 g

# Chicken Omelet

Preparation time: 5 minutes

Cooking time: 15 minutes

Servings: 1

## Ingredients:

- 2 bacon slices; cooked and crumbled
- 2 eggs
- 1 tablespoon of homemade mayonnaise
- 1 tomato; chopped.
- 1-ounce of rotisserie chicken; shredded
- 1 teaspoon of mustard
- 1 small avocado; pitted, peeled and chopped.
- Salt and black pepper to the taste.

## Directions:

1. In a bowl, mix eggs with some salt and pepper and whisk gently.
2. Heat up a pan over medium heat, spray with some vegetable oil, add eggs and cook your omelet for 5

minutes. Add chicken, avocado, tomato, bacon, mayo and mustard on one half of the omelet.

3. Fold omelet, cover pan and cook for 5 minutes more.
4. Transfer to a plate and serve.


**Nutrition:**

- Calories: 400
- Fat: 32 g
- Fiber: 6 g
- Carbs: 4 g
- Protein: 25 g

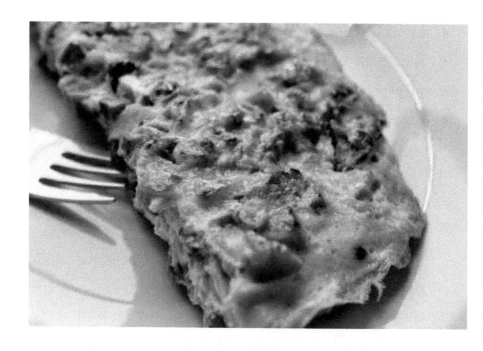

# Almond Coconut Cereal

Preparation time: 5 minutes

Cooking time: 5 minutes

Servings: 2

## Ingredients:

- 1/3 cup of Water.
- 1/3 cup of Coconut milk.
- 2 tbsps. of Roasted sunflower seeds.
- 1 tbsp. of Chia seeds.
- ½ cup of Blueberries.
- 2 tbsps. of Chopped almonds.

## Directions:

1. Put a medium bowl in position and add coconut milk and chia seeds, then put aside for 5 minutes.
2. Blend almond with sunflower seeds, then add the mixture to the chia seeds mixture and add water to make them mix evenly.
3. Serve topped with the remaining sunflower seeds and blueberries.

## Nutrition:

- Calories: 181
- Fat: 15.2 g
- Fiber: 4 g
- Carbs: 10.8 g
- Protein: 3.7 g

# WW Salad in a Jar

Preparation time: 10 minutes

Cooking time: 5 minutes

Servings: 1

## Ingredients:

- 1-ounce of favorite greens
- 1-ounce of red bell pepper; chopped.
- 4 ounces' of rotisserie chicken; roughly chopped.
- 4 tablespoons of extra virgin olive oil
- 1/2 scallion; chopped.
- 1-ounce of cucumber; chopped.
- 1-ounce of cherry tomatoes; halved
- Salt and black pepper to taste.

## Directions:

1. In a bowl, mix greens with red bell pepper, tomatoes, scallion, cucumber, salt, pepper, olive oil, and toss to coat well.
2. Transfer this to a jar, top with chicken pieces and serve for breakfast.

**Nutrition:**

- Calories: 180
- Fat: 12 g
- Fiber: 4 g
- Carbs: 5 g
- Protein: 17 g

# Almond Porridge

Preparation time: 10 minutes

Cooking time: 5 minutes

Servings: 1

## Ingredients:

- ¼ tsp. of Ground cloves.
- ¼ tsp. of Nutmeg.
- 1 tsp. of Stevia.
- ¾ cup of Coconut cream.
- ½ cup of Ground almonds.
- ¼ tsp. of Ground cardamom.
- 1 tsp. of Ground cinnamon.

## Directions:

1. Set your pan over medium heat to cook the coconut milk for a couple of minutes
2. Stir in almonds and stevia to cook for 5 minutes
3. Mix in nutmeg, cardamom, and cinnamon.
4. Enjoy while still hot.

**Nutrition:**

- Calories: 695
- Fat: 66.7 g
- Fiber: 11.1 g
- Carbs: 22 g
- Protein: 14.3 g

# Special Almond Cereal

Preparation time: 5 minutes

Cooking time: 5 minutes

Servings: 1

## Ingredients:

- 2 tablespoons of almonds; chopped.
- 1/3 cup of coconut milk
- 1 tablespoon of chia seeds
- 2 tablespoon of pepitas; roasted
- A handful blueberries
- 1 small banana; chopped.
- 1/3 cup of water

## Directions:

1. In a bowl, mix chia seeds with coconut milk and leave aside for 5 minutes. In your food processor, mix half the pepitas with almonds and pulse them well.
2. Add this to chia seeds mix.
3. Also add the water and stir.

4. Top with the rest of the pepitas, banana pieces, blueberries, and serve.

## Nutrition:

- Calories: 200
- Fat: 3 g
- Fiber: 2 g
- Carbs: 5 g
- Protein: 4 g

# Bacon and Lemon spiced Muffins

Preparation time: 10 minutes

Cooking time: 20 minutes

Servings: 12

## Ingredients:

- 2 tsps. of Lemon thyme.
- Salt
- 3 cup of Almond flour.
- ½ cup of Melted butter.
- 1 tsp. of Baking soda.
- Black pepper
- 1 cup of Medium eggs.
- 4 Diced bacon.

## Directions:

1. Set a bowl in place and mix the eggs and baking soda very well. Whisk in the seasonings, butter, bacon, and lemon thyme. Set the mixture in a well-lined muffin pan.
2. Set the oven for 20 minutes at 3500 F, and allow to bake.
3. Allow the muffins to chill before serving.

**Nutrition:**

- Calories: 186
- Fat: 17.1 g
- Fiber: 0.8 g
- Carbs: 1.8 g
- Protein: 7.4 g

# Vitamin C Smoothie Cubes

Preparation time: 5 minutes

Cooking time: 8 hours to chill

Servings: 1

## Ingredients:

- 1/8 large papaya
- 1/8 mango
- 1/4 cups of chopped pineapple; fresh or frozen
- 1/8 cup of raw cauliflower florets; fresh or frozen
- 1/4 large navel oranges; peeled and halved
- 1/4 large orange bell pepper stemmed, seeded, and coarsely chopped

## Directions:

1. Halve the papaya and mango, remove the pits, and scoop their soft flesh into a high-speed blender.
2. Add the pineapple, cauliflower, oranges, and bell pepper. Blend until smooth.

3. Evenly divide the puree between 2 (16-compartment) cube trays and place them on a level surface in your freezer. Freeze for a minimum of 8 hours.
4. The cubes are often left in the cube trays until use or transferred to a freezer bag. The frozen cubes are good for about three weeks in a standard freezer, or up to six months in a chest freezer.

**Nutrition:**

- Calories: 96
- Fat: 1 g
- Protein: 2 g
- Carbohydrates: 24 g
- Fiber: 4 g

# Greek Style Mini Burger Pies

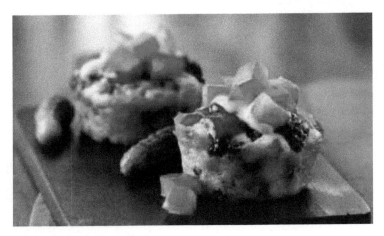

Preparation time: 15 minutes

Cooking time: 40 minutes

Servings: 6

**Ingredients:**

Burger mixture:

- Onion, large, chopped (1 piece)
- Red bell peppers, roasted, diced (1/2 cup)
- Ground lamb, 80% lean (1 pound)
- Red pepper flakes (1/4 teaspoon) Feta cheese, crumbled (2 ounces)

Baking mixture:

- Milk (1/2 cup)

- Biscuit mix, classic (1/2 cup)
- Eggs (2 pieces)

## Directions:

1. Preheat oven at 3500 F.
2. Grease 12 muffin cups using cooking spray.
3. Cook the onion and beef in a skillet heated on medium-high. Once beef is browned and cooked through, drain and allow to cool for 5 minutes. Stir with feta cheese, roasted red peppers, and red pepper flakes.
4. Whisk the baking mixture Ingredients together. Fill each muffin cup with baking mixture (1 tablespoon).
5. Air-fry for twenty-five to thirty minutes. Let cool before serving.

## Nutrition:

- Calories 270
- Fat: 10 g
- Protein: 10 g
- Carbohydrates: 10 g

# Awesome Avocado Muffins

Preparation time: 10 minutes

Cooking time: 20 minutes

Servings: 12

## Ingredients:

- 6 bacon slices; chopped.
- 1 yellow onion; chopped.
- 1/2 teaspoon of baking soda
- 1/2 cup of coconut flour
- 1 cup of coconut milk
- 2 cups of avocado; pitted, peeled and chopped.
- 4 eggs
- Salt and black pepper to taste.

## Directions:

1. Heat up a pan, add onion and bacon; stir and brown for a couple of minutes. In a bowl, mash avocado pieces with a fork and whisk well with the eggs. Add milk, salt, pepper, baking soda, coconut flour, and stir everything.
2. Add bacon mix and stir again.

3. Add coconut oil to muffin tray, divide eggs and avocado mix into the tray, heat oven at 3500 F and bake for 20 minutes
4. Divide muffins between plates and serve them for breakfast.

**Nutrition:**

- Calories: 200
- Fat: 7 g
- Fiber: 4 g
- Carbs: 7 g
- Protein: 5 g

# Raw-Cinnamon-Apple Nut Bowl

Preparation time: 15 minutes

Cooking time: 1 hour to chill

Servings: 1

## Ingredients:

- One green apple; halved, seeded, and cored
- 3/4 Honeycrisp apples; halved, seeded, and cored
- 1/4 teaspoon of freshly squeezed lemon juice
- One pitted Medrol dates
- 1/8 teaspoon of ground cinnamon
- Pinch of ground nutmeg
- 1/2 tablespoons of chia seeds, plus more for serving (optional)
- 1/4 tablespoon of hemp seed
- 1/8 cup of chopped walnuts Nut butter, for serving (optional)

## Directions:

1. Finely dice half the green apple and one candy apple. Mix with the lemon juice and store in an airtight container while you are executing subsequent steps.
2. Coarsely chop the remaining apples and the dates. Transfer to a food processor and add the cinnamon and nutmeg.
3. Check it several times to see if it's mixing, then process for 2 to 3 minutes to puree. Stir the puree into the reserved diced apples.
4. Stir in the chia seeds (if using), hemp seeds, and walnuts.
5. Chill for a minimum of one hour.
6. Enjoy!
7. Serve as it is or top with additional chia seeds and spread (if using).

## Nutrition:

- Calories: 274
- Fat: 8 g
- Protein: 4 g
- Carbohydrates: 52 g
- Fiber: 9 g

# Family Fun Pizza

Preparation time: 30 minutes

Cooking time: 25 minutes

Servings: 16

## Ingredients:

Pizza crust:

- Water; warm (1 cup)
- Salt (1/2 teaspoon)
- Flour, whole wheat (1 cup)
- Olive oil (2 tablespoons)
- Dry yeast; quick active (1 package)
- Flour, all purpose (1 ½ cups)
- Cornmeal
- Olive oil

Filling:

- Onion; chopped (1 cup)
- Mushrooms; sliced, drained (4 ounces)
- Garlic cloves; chopped finely (2 pieces)
- Parmesan cheese; grated (1/4 cup)
- Ground lamb; 80% lean (1 pound)

- Italian seasoning (1 teaspoon)
- Pizza sauce (8 ounces)
- Mozzarella cheese; shredded (2 cups)

## Directions:

1. Mix yeast with warm water. Combine with flours, oil (2 tablespoons), and salt by stirring then beating vigorously for half a minute. Let the dough sit for twenty minutes.
2. Preheat oven at 3500 F.
3. Prep 2 square pans (8-inch) by greasing with oil and then sprinkling with cornmeal.
4. Cut the rested dough in half; place each half inside each pan. Set aside, covered, for 30 to 45 minutes. Cook in the air fryer for 20 to 22 minutes.
5. Sauté the onion, beef, garlic, and Italian seasoning until beef is totally cooked. Drain and put aside.
6. Cover the air-fried crusts with pizza sauce before topping with beef mixture, cheeses, and mushrooms.
7. Return to oven and cook for 20 minutes.

## Nutrition:

- Calories 215
- Fat 0 g
- Protein 10 g
- Carbohydrates 20.0 g

# Tasty WW Pancakes

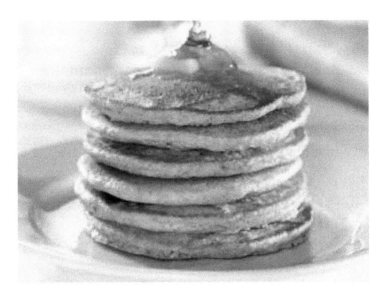

Preparation time: 12 minutes

Cooking time: 3 minutes

Servings: 4


**Ingredients:**

- 2 ounces of cream cheese
- 1 teaspoon of stevia
- 1/2 teaspoon of cinnamon; ground
- 2 eggs
- Cooking spray

## Directions:

1. Mix the eggs with the cream cheese, stevia, and cinnamon in a blender, and blend well.
2. Heat pan with cooking spray over medium-high heat. Add 1/4 of the batter, spread well, cook for 2 minutes, invert and cook for 1 minute more.
3. Move to a plate and repeat the process with the rest of the dough.
4. Serve them directly.

## Nutrition:

- Calories: 344
- Fat: 23 g
- Fiber: 12 g
- Carbs: 3 g
- Protein: 16 g

# Slow Cooker Savory Butternut Squash Oatmeal

Preparation time: 15 minutes

Cooking time: 6 to 8 hours

Servings: 1

## Ingredients:

- 1/4 cup of steel-cut oats
- 1/2 cups of cubed (1/2-inch pieces), peeled butternut squash (after preparing a whole squash, freeze any leftovers for future meals)
- 3/4 cups of water
- 1/16 cup of unsweetened nondairy milk
- 1/4 tablespoon of chia seeds
- 1/2 teaspoons of yellow miso paste
- 3/4 teaspoons of ground ginger
- 1/4 tablespoon of sesame seeds; toasted
- 1/4 tablespoon of chopped scallion; green parts only
- Shredded carrot, for serving (optional)

## Directions:

1. In a slow cooker, mix the oats, butternut squash, and water.
2. Cover the slow cooker and cook on low for 6 to 8 hours, or until the squash is fork-tender.
3. Using a potato masher or heavy spoon, roughly mash the cooked butternut squash.
4. Stir to mix with the oats.
5. Whisk together the milk, chia seeds, miso paste, and ginger in a large bowl. Stir the mixture into the oats.
6. Top your oatmeal bowl with sesame seeds and scallion for more plant-based fiber, and top with shredded carrot (if using).

## Nutrition:

- Calories: 230
- Fat: 5 g
- Protein: 7 g
- Carbohydrates: 40 g
- Fiber: 9 g

# Yummy Smoked Salmon

Preparation time: 10 minutes

Cooking time: 10 minutes

Servings: 3

## Ingredients:

- 4 eggs; whisked
- 1/2 teaspoon of avocado oil
- 4 ounces of smoked salmon; chopped.
- For the sauce:
- 1/2 cup of cashews; soaked and drained
- 1/4 cup of green onions; chopped.
- 1 teaspoon of garlic powder
- 1 cup of coconut milk
- 1 tablespoon of lemon juice
- Salt and black pepper to taste.

## Directions:

1. In your blender, mix cashews with coconut milk, garlic powder, juice, and blend well.

2. Add salt, pepper, green onions, and blend well again. Transfer to a bowl and keep in the fridge for now. Heat up a pan with the oil over medium-low heat; add eggs, whisk a touch and cook until it is almost done. Pour in your preheated broiler and cook until eggs set.
3. Divide eggs on plates, top with salmon and serve with the scallion sauce on top.

## Nutrition:

- Calories: 200
- Fat: 10 g
- Fiber: 2 g
- Carbs: 11 g
- Protein: 15 g

# Spiced Sorghum and Berries

Preparation time: 5 minutes

Cooking time: 1 hour

Servings: 1

## Ingredients:

- 1/4 cup of whole-grain sorghum
- 1/4 teaspoon of ground cinnamon
- 1/4 teaspoon of Chinese five-spice powder
- 3/4 cups of water
- 1/4 cup of unsweetened nondairy milk
- 1/4 teaspoon of vanilla extract
- 1/2 tablespoons of pure maple syrup
- 1/2 tablespoon of chia seed
- 1/8 cup of sliced almonds
- 1/2 cups of fresh raspberries; divided

## Directions:

1. Place a large pot over medium-high heat, stir in together the sorghum, cinnamon, five-spice powder, and water.

2. Wait for the water to boil, cover it, and reduce the heat to medium-low.

3. Cook for 1 hour, or until the sorghum is soft and chewy. If the sorghum grains are still hard, add another cup of water and cook for 15 minutes more.

4. Using a glass cup, whisk together the milk, vanilla, and syrup to blend.

5. Add the mixture to the sorghum and the chia seeds, almonds, and 1 cup of raspberries. Gently stir to mix.

6. When serving, top with the remaining one cup of fresh raspberries.

**Nutrition:**

- Calories: 289
- Fat: 8 g
- Protein: 9 g
- Carbohydrates: 52 g
- Fiber: 10 g

# WW Breakfast Cereal

Preparation time: 10 minutes

Cooking time: 3 minutes

Servings: 2

## Ingredients:

- 1/2 cup of coconut; shredded
- 1/3 cup of macadamia nuts; chopped.
- 4 teaspoons of ghee
- 2 cups of almond milk
- 1 tablespoon of stevia
- 1/3 cup of walnuts; chopped
- 1/3 cup of flax seed
- A pinch of salt

## Directions:

1. Heat a pot of mistletoe over medium heat. Add the milk, coconut, salt, macadamia nuts, walnuts, flax seeds, stevia, and blend well.
2. Cook for 3 minutes. Stir again, and remove from heat for 10 minutes.

3.  Divide into 2 bowls and serve

## Nutrition:

- Calories: 140
- Fat: 3 g
- Fiber: 2 g
- Carbs: 1. 5 g
- Protein: 7 g

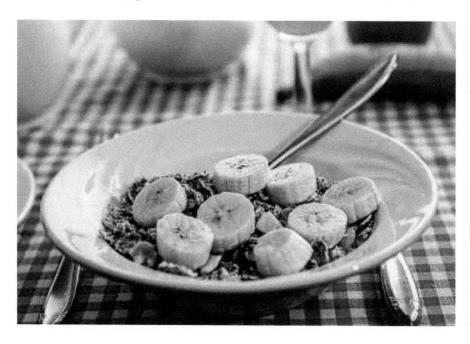

# Asparagus Frittata Recipe

Preparation time: 20 minutes

Cooking time: 20 minutes

Servings: 4

## Ingredients:

- 4 Bacon slices; chopped
- Salt and black pepper
- 8 Eggs; whisked
- 1 bunch of asparagus; trimmed and chopped

## Directions:

1. Heat a pan, add bacon, stir and cook for 5 minutes.
2. Add asparagus, salt, and pepper, stir and cook for an additional 5 minutes.
3. Add the chilled eggs, spread them in the pan, allow them to substitute the oven and bake for 20 minutes at 350°F.
4. Share and divide between plates and serve for breakfast.

**Nutrition:**

- Calories: 251
- Carbs: 16 g
- Fat: 6 g
- Fiber: 8 g
- Protein: 7 g

# Avocados Stuffed with Salmon

Preparation time: 5 minutes

Cooking time: 5 minutes

Servings: 2

## Ingredients:

- 1 Avocado; pitted and halved
- 2 tablespoons of olive oil
- 1 Lemon juice
- 2 ounces of Smoked salmon; flaked
- 1 ounce of Goat cheese; crumbled
- Salt and black pepper

## Directions:

1. Mix the salmon with lemon juice, olive oil, cheese, salt, and pepper in your food processor and pulsate well.
2. Divide this mixture into avocado halves and serve.
3. Dish and Enjoy!

**Nutrition:**

- Calories: 300
- Fat: 15 g
- Fiber: 5 g
- Carbs: 8 g
- Protein: 16 g

# Tropical Greens Smoothie

Preparation time: 5 Minutes

Cooking time: 0 Minutes

Servings: 1

## Ingredients:

- 1 banana
- 1/2 large navel orange; peeled and segmented
- 1/2 cup of frozen mango chunks
- 1 cup of frozen spinach
- 1 celery stalk; broken into pieces
- 1 tablespoon of cashew butter or almond butter
- 1/2 tablespoon of spiraling
- 1/2 tablespoon of ground flaxseed
- 1/2 cup of unsweetened nondairy milk
- Water; for thinning (optional)

## Directions:

1. In a high-speed blender or food processor, mix the bananas, orange, mango, spinach, celery, cashew butter, spiraling (if using), flaxseed, and milk.

2. Blend until creamy, adding more milk or water to thin the smoothie if too thick. Serve immediately—it is best served fresh.

**Nutrition:**

- Calories: 391
- Fat: 12 g
- Protein: 13 g
- Carbohydrates: 68 g
- Fiber: 13 g

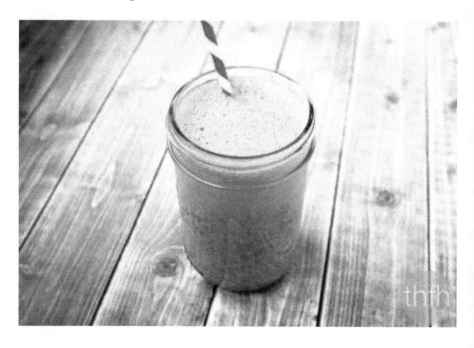

# Overnight Chocolate Chia Pudding

Preparation time: 2 minutes

Cooking time: overnight to chill

Servings: 1

**Ingredients:**

- 1/8 cup of chia seeds
- 1/2 cup of unsweetened nondairy milk
- 1 tablespoon of raw cocoa powder
- 1/2 teaspoon of vanilla extract
- 1/2 teaspoon of pure maple syrup

**Directions:**

1. Mix together the chia seeds, milk, cacao powder, vanilla, and syrup in a large bowl.
2. Divide between two (1/2-pint) covered glass jars or containers.
3. Refrigerate overnight.
4. Stir before serving.

**Nutrition:**

- Calories: 213
- Fat: 10 g
- Protein: 9 g
- Carbohydrates: 20 g
- Fiber: 15 g

# Carrot Cake Oatmeal

Preparation time: 10 minutes

Cooking time: 15 minutes

Servings: 1

## Ingredients:

- 1/8 cup of pecans
- 1/2 cup of finely shredded carrot
- 1/4 cup of old-fashioned oats
- 5/8 cups of unsweetened nondairy milk
- 1/2 tablespoon of pure maple syrup
- 1/2 teaspoon of ground cinnamon
- 1/2 teaspoon of ground ginger
- 1/8 teaspoon of ground nutmeg
- 1 tablespoon of chia seed

## Directions:

1. Over medium-high heat in a skillet, toast the pecans for 3 to 4 minutes, often stirring, until browned and fragrant (watch closely, as they will burn quickly).

2. Pour the pecans onto a chopping board and coarsely chop them. Set aside.
3. In an 8-quart pot over medium-high heat, mix the carrot, oats, milk, maple syrup, cinnamon, ginger, and nutmeg.
4. When it has started boiling, reduce the heat to medium-low.
5. Cook, uncovered, for 10 minutes, stirring occasionally.
6. Stir in the chopped pecans and chia seeds. Serve immediately.

## Nutrition:

- Calories: 307
- Fat: 17 g
- Protein: 7 g
- Carbohydrates: 35 g
- Fiber: 11 g

# Bacon Spaghetti Squash Carbonara

Preparation time: 20 minutes

Cooking time: 40 minutes

Servings: 4

## Ingredients:

- 1 small spaghetti squash
- 6 ounces of bacon (roughly chopped)
- 1 large tomato; sliced
- 2 chives; chopped
- 1 garlic clove; minced
- 6 ounces of low-fat cottage cheese
- 1 cup of Gouda cheese; grated
- 2 tablespoons of olive oil
- Salt and pepper, to taste

## Directions:

1. Preheat the oven to 350°F.

2. Cut the squash spaghetti in half, brush with some vegetable oil and bake for 20–30 minutes, skin side up. Remove from the oven and take away the core with a fork, creating the spaghetti.

3. Heat one tablespoon of olive oil in a skillet. Cook the bacon for about 1 minute until crispy.

4. Quickly wipe out the pan with paper towels.

5. Heat another tablespoon of oil and sauté the garlic, tomato, and chives for 2–3 minutes. Add the spaghetti and sauté for an additional 5 minutes, occasionally stirring to keep from burning.

6. Start putting in the pot cheese, about 2 tablespoons at a time. If the sauce becomes thick, add a few cups of water. The sauce should be creamy but not too runny or thick. Allow to cook for an additional 3 minutes.

7. Serve immediately.

**Nutrition:**

- Calories: 305
- Total Fat: 21 g
- Net Carbs: 8 g
- Protein: 18 g

# Vanilla Buckwheat Porridge

Preparation time: 5 minutes

Cooking time: 25 minutes

Servings: 1

## Ingredients:

- 1 cup of water
- 1/4 cup of raw buckwheat grouts
- 1/4 teaspoon of ground cinnamon
- 1/4 banana; sliced
- 1/16 cup of golden raisins
- 1/16 cup of dried currants
- 1/16 cup of sunflower seeds
- 1/2 tablespoons of chia seeds
- 1/4 tablespoon of hemp seeds
- 1/4 tablespoon of sesame seeds, toasted
- 1/8 cup of unsweetened nondairy milk
- 1/4 tablespoon of pure maple syrup
- 1/4 teaspoon of vanilla extract

## Directions:

1. Boil the water in a pot. Stir in the buckwheat, cinnamon, and banana.
2. Cook the mixture and wait for it to boil, then reduce the heat to medium-low.
3. Cover the pot and cook for 15 minutes, or until the buckwheat is soft and then remove from the heat.
4. Stir in the raisins, currants, sunflower seeds, chia seeds, hemp seeds, sesame seeds, milk, maple syrup, and vanilla. Cover the pot. Wait for 10 minutes before serving.
5. Serve as it is or top as desired.

## Nutrition:

- Calories: 353
- Fat: 11 g
- Protein: 10 g
- Carbohydrates: 61 g
- Fiber: 10 g

# Broccoli with Bell Peppers

Servings: 6

Preparation time: 10 minutes

Cooking time: 10 minutes

## Ingredients:

- 2 tablespoons of olive oil
- 4 garlic cloves, minced
- 1 large white onion, sliced
- 2 cups of small broccoli florets
- 3 red bell peppers, seeded and sliced
- ¼ cup of low-sodium vegetable broth
- Salt and ground black pepper, as required

## Instructions:

1. In a large wok, heat oil over medium heat and sauté the garlic for about 1 minute.
2. Add the onion, broccoli and bell peppers and cook for about 5 minutes, stirring frequently.
3. Stir in the broth and cook for about 4 minutes, stirring frequently.

4. Stir in the salt and black pepper and take away from the heat.
5. Serve hot.

# Stuffed Zucchini

Servings: 8

Preparation time: 15 minutes

Cooking time: 18 minutes

## Ingredients:

- 4 medium zucchinis, halved lengthwise
- 1 cup of red bell pepper, seeded and minced
- ½ cup of Kalamata olives, pitted and minced
- ½ cup of tomatoes, minced
- 1 teaspoon of garlic, minced
- 1 tablespoon of dried oregano, crushed
- Salt and ground black pepper, as required
- ½ cup of feta cheese, crumbled
- ¼ cup of fresh parsley, chopped finely

## Instructions:

1. Preheat your oven to 350 degrees F.
2. Grease a large baking sheet.
3. With a melon baller, scoop out the flesh of every zucchini half. Discard the flesh.

4. In a bowl, mix bell pepper, olives, tomato, garlic, oregano and black pepper.
5. Stuff each zucchini half with the veggie mixture evenly.
6. Arrange zucchini halves onto the prepared baking sheet and Bake for about 15 minutes.
7. Now, set the oven to broiler on high.
8. Top each zucchini half with feta cheese and broil for about 3 minutes.
9. Garnish with parsley and serve hot.

# Zucchini & Bell Pepper Curry

Servings: 6

Preparation time: 20 minutes

Cooking time: 20 minutes

## Ingredients:

- 2 medium zucchinis, chopped
- 1 green bell pepper, seeded and cubed
- 1 red bell pepper, seeded and cubed
- 1 yellow onion, sliced thinly
- 2 tablespoons of olive oil
- 2 teaspoons of curry powder
- Salt and ground black pepper, as required
- ¼ cup of homemade low-sodium vegetable broth
- ¼ cup of fresh cilantro, chopped

## Instructions:

1. Preheat your oven to 375 degrees F.
2. Lightly grease a large baking dish.
3. In a large bowl, add all Ingredients except cilantro and blend until well combined.

4. Transfer the vegetable mixture into prepared baking dish.

5. Bake for about 15-20 minutes.

6. Serve immediately with the garnishing of cilantro

# Zucchini Noodles with Mushroom Sauce

Servings: 5

Preparation time: 20 minutes

Cooking time: 15 minutes

## Ingredients:

For Mushroom Sauce:

- 1½ tablespoons of olive oil
- 1 large garlic clove, minced
- 1¼ cups of fresh button mushrooms, sliced
- ¼ cup of homemade low-sodium vegetable broth
- ¼ cup of cream
- Salt and ground black pepper, as to require

For Zucchini Noodles:

- 3 large zucchinis, spiralized with blade C
- ¼ cup of fresh parsley leaves, chopped

## Instructions:

1. For mushroom sauce: In a large skillet, heat the oil over medium heat and sauté the garlic for about 1 minute.
2. Stir in the mushrooms and cook for about 6-8 minutes.
3. Stir in the broth and cook for about 2 minutes, stirring continuously.
4. Stir in the cream, salt and black pepper and cook for about 1 minute.
5. Meanwhile, for the zucchini noodles: In a large pan of the boiling water, add the zucchini noodles and cook for about 2-3 minutes.
6. With a slotted spoon, transfer the zucchini noodles into a colander and immediately rinse under cold running water.
7. Drain the zucchini noodles well and transfer onto a large paper towel-lined plate to drain.
8. Divide the zucchini noodles onto serving plates evenly.
9. Remove the sauce from the heat and place over zucchini noodles evenly.
10. Serve immediately with the garnishing of parsley.

# Squash Casserole

Servings: 8

Preparation time: 15 minutes

Cooking time: 55 minutes

## Ingredients:

- ¼ cup of plus 2 tablespoons of olive oil, divided
- 1 small yellow onion, chopped
- 3 summer squashes, sliced
- 4 eggs, beaten
- 3 cups of low-fat cheddar cheese, shredded and divided
- 2 tablespoons of unsweetened almond milk
- 2-3 tablespoons of almond flour
- 2 tablespoons of Erythritol
- Salt and ground black pepper, as required

## Instructions:

1. Preheat the oven to 375 degrees F.
2. In a large skillet, heat 2 tablespoons of oil over medium heat and cook the onion and squash for about 8-10 minutes, stirring occasionally.

3. Remove the skillet from the heat.

4. Place the eggs, 1 cup of cheddar cheese, almond milk, almond flour, Erythritol, salt and black pepper in a large bowl and blend until well combined.

5. Add the squash mixture, and remaining oil and stir to mix.

6. Transfer the mixture into a large casserole dish and sprinkle with the remaining cheddar cheese.

7. Bake for about 35-45 minutes.

8. Remove the casserole dish from oven and put aside for about 5-10 minutes before serving.

9. Cut into 8 equal-sized portions and serve.

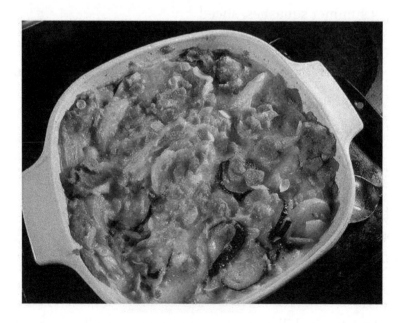

# Veggies & Walnut Loaf

Servings: 10

Preparation time: 15 minutes

Cooking time: 1 hour 10 minutes

## Ingredients:

- 1 tablespoon of olive oil
- 2 yellow onions, chopped
- 2 garlic cloves, minced
- 1 teaspoon of dried rosemary, crushed1 cup of walnuts, chopped
- 2 large carrots, peeled and chopped
- 1 large celery stalk, chopped
- 1 large green bell pepper, seeded and chopped
- 1 cup of fresh button mushrooms, chopped
- 5 large eggs
- 1¼ cups of almond flour
- Salt and ground black pepper, to taste

## Instructions:

1. Preheat your oven to 350-degree F.

2. Line 2 loaf pans with lightly greased parchment papers.

3. In a large wok, heat the vegetable oil over medium heat and sauté the onion for about 4-5 minutes.

4. Add the garlic and rosemary and sauté for about 1 minute.

5. Add the walnuts and vegetables and cook for about 3–4 minutes.

6. Remove the wok from heat and transfer the mixture into a large bowl.

7. Put aside to chill slightly.

8. In another bowl, add the eggs, flour, sea salt, and black pepper, and beat until well combined.

9. Add the egg mixture into the bowl with vegetable mixture and blend until well combined.

10. Divide the mixture into prepared loaf pans evenly.

11. Bake for about 50–60 minutes or until the top becomes golden brown.

12. Remove from the oven and put aside to chill slightly.

13. Carefully invert the loaves onto a platter.

14. Cut into desired sized slices and serve.

# Tofu & Veggie Burgers

Servings: 2

Preparation time: 20 minutes

Cooking time: 8 minutes

**Ingredients:**

For Patties:

- ½ cup of firm tofu pressed and drained
- 1 medium carrot, peeled and gated
- 1 tablespoon of onion, chopped
- 1 tablespoon of scallion, chopped
- 1 tablespoon of fresh parsley, chopped
- ½ garlic clove, minced
- 2 teaspoons of low-sodium soy sauce
- 1 tablespoon of arrowroot flour
- 1 teaspoon of Nutritional yeast flakes
- ½ teaspoon of Dijon mustard
- 1 teaspoon of paprika
- ¼ teaspoon of ground turmeric
- ½ teaspoon of ground black pepper
- 2 tablespoons of olive oil

For Serving:

- ½ cup of cherry tomatoes halved
- 2 cup of fresh baby greens

## Instructions:

1. For patties: in a bowl, add the tofu and with a fork, mash well.
2. Add the remaining Ingredients apart from oil and blend until well combined.
3. Make 4 equal-sized patties from the mixture.
4. Heat the oil in a frying pan over low heat and cook the patties for about 4 minutes per side.
5. Divide the avocado, tomatoes and greens onto serving plates.
6. Top each plate with 2 patties and serve.

# Tofu & Veggie Lettuce Wraps

Servings: 4

Preparation time: 15 minutes

Cooking time: 6 minutes

**Ingredients:**

For Wraps:

- 1 tablespoon of olive oil
- 14 ounces of extra-firm tofu, drained, pressed and cut into cubes
- 1 teaspoon of curry powder
- Salt, as required
- 8 lettuce leaves
- 1 small carrot, peeled and julienned
- ½ cup of radishes, sliced
- 2 tablespoons of fresh cilantro, chopped

For Sauce:

- ½ cup of creamy peanut butter
- 1 tablespoon of maple syrup
- 2 tablespoons of low-sodium soy sauce
- 2 tablespoons of fresh lime juice

- ¼ teaspoon of red pepper flakes, crushed
- ¼ cup of water

## Instructions:

1. For tofu: in a skillet, heat the oil over medium heat and cook the tofu, curry powder and a little salt for about 5-6 minutes or until golden brown, stirring frequently.
2. Remove from the heat and put aside to chill slightly.
3. Meanwhile, for sauce: in a bowl, add all the Ingredients and beat until smooth.
4. Arrange the lettuce leaves onto serving plates.
5. Divide the tofu, carrot, radish and peanuts over each leaf evenly.
6. Garnish with cilantro and serve alongside the peanut sauce.

# Tofu with Kale

Servings: 2

Preparation time: 15 minutes

Cooking time: 10 minutes

## Ingredients:

- 1 tablespoon of extra-virgin olive oil
- ½ pound tofu, pressed, drained and cubed
- 1 teaspoon of fresh ginger, minced
- 1 garlic clove, minced
- ¼ teaspoon of red pepper flakes, crushed
- 6 ounces of fresh kale, tough ribs removed and chopped finely
- 1 tablespoon of low-sodium soy sauce

## Instructions:

1. In a large non-stick wok, heat vegetable oil over medium-high heat and stir-fry the tofu for about 3-3 minutes.
2. Add the ginger, garlic and red pepper flakes and cook for about 1 minute, stirring continuously.
3. Stir in the kale and soy and stir-fry for about 4-5 minutes.
4. Serve hot.

# Tofu with Broccoli

Servings: 4

Preparation time: 20 minutes

Cooking time: 25 minutes

## Ingredients:

For Tofu:

- 14 ounces of firm tofu, drained, pressed and cut into 1-inch slices
- 1/3 cup of arrowroot starch, divided
- ¼ cup of olive oil
- 1 teaspoon of fresh ginger, grated
- 1 medium onion, sliced thinly
- 3 tablespoons of low-sodium soy sauce
- 2 tablespoons of balsamic vinegar
- 1 tablespoon of maple syrup
- ½ cup of water

For Steamed Broccoli:

- 2 cups of broccoli florets

## Instructions:

1. In a shallow bowl, place ¼ cup of the arrowroot starch.
2. Add the tofu cubes and coat with arrowroot starch.
3. In a cast-iron wok, heat the vegetable oil over medium heat and cook the tofu cubes for about 8-10 minutes or until golden from all sides.
4. With a slotted spoon, transfer the tofu cubes onto a plate. Set aside.
5. In the same wok, add ginger and sauté for about 1 minute.
6. Add the onions and sauté for about 2-3 minutes.
7. Add the soy sauce, vinegar and syrup and bring to a mild simmer.
8. In the meantime, in a small bowl, dissolve the remaining arrowroot starch in water.
9. Slowly, add the arrowroot starch mixture into the sauce, stirring continuously.
10. Stir in the cooked tofu and cook for about 1 minute.
11. Meanwhile, in a large pan of water, arrange a steamer basket and bring to a boil.
12. Adjust the heat to medium-low.
13. Place the broccoli florets in the steamer basket and steam, covered for about 5-6 minutes.
14. Remove from the heat and drain the broccoli completely.
15. Transfer the broccoli into the wok of tofu and stir to mix.
16. Serve hot.

# Tofu with Peas

Servings: 5

Preparation time: 15 minutes

Cooking time: 20 minutes

## Ingredients:

- 2 tablespoons of olive oil, divided
- 1 (16-ounce of) package extra-firm tofu, drained, pressed and cubed
- 1 cup of yellow onion, chopped
- 1 tablespoon of fresh ginger, minced
- 2 garlic cloves, minced
- 1 tomato, chopped finely
- 2 cups of frozen peas, thawed
- ¼ cup of water
- 2 tablespoons of fresh cilantro, chopped

## Instructions:

1. In a non-stick wok, heat 1 tablespoon of the oil over medium-high heat and cook the tofu for about 4-5 minutes or until brown completely, stirring occasionally.
2. Transfer the tofu into a bowl.
3. In the same wok, heat the remaining oil over medium heat and sauté the onion for about 3-4 minutes.
4. Add the ginger and garlic and sauté for about 1 minute.
5. Add the tomatoes and cook for about 4-5 minutes, crushing with the rear of a spoon.
6. Stir in the peas and broth and cook for about 2-3 minutes.
7. Stir in the tofu and cook for about 1-2 minutes.
8. Serve hot with the garnishing of cilantro.

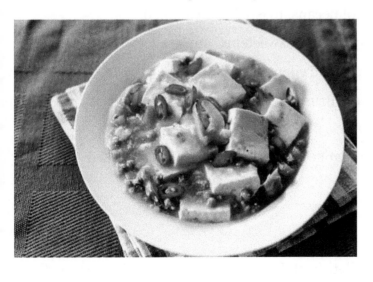

# Tofu with Brussels Sprout

Servings: 3

Preparation time: 15 minutes

Cooking time: 15 minutes

## Ingredients:

- 1½ tablespoons of olive oil, divided
- 8 ounces of extra-firm tofu, drained, pressed and cut into slices
- 2 garlic cloves, chopped
- 1/3 cup of pecans, toasted and chopped
- 1 tablespoon of unsweetened applesauce
- ¼ cup of fresh cilantro, chopped
- ½ pound Brussels sprouts, trimmed and cut into wide ribbons
- ¾ pound mixed bell peppers, seeded and sliced

## Instructions:

1. In a skillet, heat ½ tablespoon of the oil over medium heat and sauté the tofu for about 6-7 minutes or until golden brown.

2. Add the garlic and pecans and sauté for about 1 minute.
3. Add the applesauce and cook for about 2 minutes.
4. Stir in the cilantro and take away from heat.
5. Transfer tofu into a plate and put aside
6. In the same skillet, heat the remaining oil over medium-high heat and cook the Brussels sprouts and bell peppers for about 5 minutes.
7. Stir in the tofu and take away from the heat.
8. Serve immediately.

# Tofu with Veggies

Servings: 4

Preparation time: 20 minutes

Cooking time: 45 minutes

## Ingredients:

- 1 (14-ounce of) package extra-firm tofu, pressed, drained and cut into small cubes
- 2 tablespoons of sesame oil, divided
- 4 tablespoons of low-sodium soy sauce
- 3 tablespoons of maple syrup
- 2 tablespoons of peanut butter
- 2 tablespoons of fresh lime juice
- 1-2 teaspoons of chili garlic sauce
- 1-pound green beans, trimmed
- 2-3 small red bell peppers, seeded and cubed
- 2 scallion greens, chopped

## Instructions:

1. Preheat your oven to 400 degrees F.
2. Line a baking sheet with parchment paper.

3. Arrange the tofu cubes onto the prepared baking sheet in a single layer.

4. Bake for about 25-30 minutes.

5. Meanwhile, in a small bowl, add 1 tablespoon of the olive oil, soy sauce, maple syrup, spread, lemon juice, and chili aioli and beat until well combined. Set aside.

6. Remove from the oven and place the tofu cubes into the bowl of sauce.

7. Stir the mixture well and put aside for about 10 minutes, stirring occasionally.

8. With a slotted spoon, remove the tofu cubes from the bowl, reserving the sauce.

9. Heat a large cast-iron skillet over medium heat and cook the tofu cubes for about 5 minutes, stirring occasionally.

10. With a slotted spoon, transfer the tofu cubes onto a plate. Set aside.

11. In the same skillet, add the remaining vegetable oil, green beans, bell peppers and 2-3 tablespoons of reserved sauce and cook, covered for about 4-5 minutes.

12. Adjust the heat to medium-high, and stir in the cooked tofu remaining reserved sauce.

13. Cook for about 1-2 minutes, stirring frequently.

14. Stir in the scallion greens and serve hot.

# Tofu & Mushroom Curry

Servings: 4

Preparation time: 20 minutes

Cooking time: 25 minutes

**Ingredients:**

For Tofu:

- 16 ounces of extra-firm tofu, pressed, drained and cut into ½-inch cubes
- 1 garlic clove, minced
- 3 tablespoons of balsamic vinegar
- 3 tablespoons of low-sodium soy sauce
- 3 tablespoons of arrowroot starch
- 2 tablespoons of sesame oil
- 1 tablespoon of Erythritol
- 1 teaspoon of red pepper flakes
- 2 tablespoons of coconut oil

For Curry:

- ¼ cup of water
- 1 small yellow onion, minced
- 3 large garlic cloves, minced

- 1 teaspoon of fresh ginger, grated
- 2 cups of fresh mushrooms, sliced
- 3 tablespoons of red curry paste
- 13 ounces of light coconut milk
- 1 tablespoon of low-sodium soy sauce
- 2 tablespoons of fresh lime juice
- 1 teaspoon of lime zest, grated
- 8 fresh basil leaves, chopped

## Instructions:

1. For tofu: in a resealable bag, place all Ingredients.
2. Seal the bag and shake to coat well.
3. Refrigerate to marinate for 2-4 hours.
4. In a large skillet, melt the coconut oil over medium heat and fry the tofu cubes for about 4-5 minutes or until golden brown completely.
5. With a slotted spoon, transfer the tofu cubes into a bowl.
6. For curry: in a large pan, add the water over medium heat and bring to a simmer.
7. Add the minced onion, garlic and ginger and cook for about 5 minutes.
8. Add the mushrooms and curry paste and stir to mix well.
9. Stir in the remaining Ingredients apart from basil and simmer for about 10 minutes.
10. Stir in the tofu and simmer for about 5 minutes.

11. Garnish with basil and serve.

# Tofu & Veggies Curry

Servings: 5

Preparation time: 20 minutes

Cooking time: 30 minutes

## Ingredients:

- 1 (16-ounce of) block firm tofu, drained, pressed and cut into ½-inch cubes
- 2 tablespoons of coconut oil
- 1 medium yellow onion, chopped
- 1½ tablespoons of fresh ginger, minced
- 2 garlic cloves, minced
- 1 tablespoon of curry powder
- Salt and ground black pepper, as required
- 1 cup of fresh mushrooms, sliced
- 1 cup of carrots, peeled and sliced
- 1 (14-ounce of) can unsweeten low-fat coconut milk
- ½ cup of low-sodium vegetable broth
- 2 teaspoons of Erythritol
- 10 ounces of cauliflower florets
- 1 tablespoon of fresh lime juice
- ¼ cup of fresh basil leaves, sliced thinly

**Instructions:**

1. In a Dutch oven, heat the oil over medium heat and sauté the onion, ginger and garlic for about 5 minutes.
2. Stir in the curry powder, salt and black pepper and cook for about 2 minutes, stirring occasionally.
3. Add the mushrooms and carrot and cook for about 4-5 minutes.
4. Stir in the coconut milk, broth and sugar and bring to a boil.
5. Add the tofu and cauliflower and simmer for about 12-15 minutes, stirring occasionally.
6. Stir in the juice and take away from the heat.
7. Serve hot.

# Tempeh with Bell Peppers

Servings: 3

Preparation time: 15 minutes

Cooking time: 15 minutes

## Ingredients:

- 2 tablespoons of balsamic vinegar
- 2 tablespoons of low-sodium soy sauce
- 2 tablespoons of tomato sauce
- 1 teaspoon of maple syrup
- ½ teaspoon of garlic powder
- 1/8 teaspoon of red pepper flakes, crushed
- 1 tablespoon of vegetable oil
- 8 ounces of tempeh, cut into cubes
- 1 medium onion, chopped
- 2 large green bell peppers, seeded and chopped

## Instructions:

1. In a small bowl, add the vinegar, soy sauce, spaghetti sauce, maple syrup, garlic powder and red pepper flakes and beat until well combined. Put aside.

2. Heat 1 tablespoon of oil in a large skillet over medium heat and cook the tempeh about 2-3 minutes per side.

3. Add the onion and bell peppers and heat for about 2-3 minutes.

4. Stir in the sauce mixture and cook for about 3-5 minutes, stirring frequently.

5. Serve hot.

# Tempeh with Brussel Sprout & Kale

Servings: 3

Preparation time: 15 minutes

Cooking time: 17 minutes

## Ingredients:

- 2 tablespoons of olive oil
- 1/3 cup of red onion, chopped finely
- 1½ cups of tempeh, cubed
- 2 cups of Brussels sprout, quartered
- 2 garlic cloves, minced
- ½ teaspoon of ground cumin
- ½ teaspoon of garlic powder
- Salt and ground black pepper, to taste
- 2 cups of fresh kale, tough ribs removed and chopped

## Instructions:

1. Heat the oil in a skillet over medium-high heat and sauté the onion for about 4-5 minutes.

2. Add in remaining Ingredients apart from kale and cook for about 6-7 minutes, stirring occasionally.
3. Add kale and cook for about 5 minutes, stirring twice.
4. Serve hot.

# Tempeh with Veggies

Servings: 3

Preparation time: 15 minutes

Cooking time: 17 minutes

## Ingredients:

For Sauce:

- 3 tablespoons of tahini
- 2 tablespoons of low-sodium soy sauce
- 1 tablespoon of sesame oil
- 1 tablespoon of chili garlic sauce
- 1 tablespoon of maple syrup

For tempeh & Veggies:

- 3 tablespoons of olive oil, divided
- 8 ounces of tempeh, cut into 1x2-inch rectangular strips
- 8 ounces of fresh button mushrooms, sliced thinly
- 8 ounces of fresh spinach
- 1 tablespoon of fresh ginger, minced
- 1 tablespoon of garlic, minced

**Instructions:**

1. For sauce: in a bowl, add all Ingredients and beat until well combined.
2. In a large skillet, heat the oil over medium-high heat and cook the tempeh for about 4-5 minutes or until browned.
3. With a slotted spoon, transfer the tempeh into a bowl and put aside.
4. In the same skillet, heat the remaining oil over medium-high heat and cook the mushrooms for about 6-7 minutes, stirring frequently.
5. With a slotted spoon, transfer the mushrooms into a bowl and put aside.
6. In the same skillet, add the spinach, ginger and garlic and cook for about 2-3 minutes.
7. Stir in the cooked tempeh, mushrooms and sauce and cook for about 1-2 minutes, stirring continuously.
8. Serve hot.

# Parmesan Eggs in Avocado Cup

Servings: 2

Preparation time: 10 minutes

Cooking time: 12 minutes

## Ingredients:

- 1 avocado, halved and pitted
- Salt and ground black pepper, as required
- 2 eggs
- 1 tablespoon of low-fat Parmesan cheese, shredded

## Instructions:

1. Arrange a greased square piece of foil in the air fry basket.
2. Select "Bake" of Breville Smart Air Fryer Oven and adjust the temperature to 390 degrees F.
3. Set the timer for 12 minutes and press "Start/Stop" to start preheating.
4. Meanwhile, carefully scoop out about 2 teaspoons of flesh from each avocado half.

5. Crack 1 egg in each avocado half and sprinkle with salt, black pepper and cheese.

6. When the unit beeps to point out that it's preheated, arrange the avocado halves into the prepared air fry basket and insert in the oven.

7. When the Cooking time is completed, transfer the avocado halves onto serving plates.

8. Top with Parmesan and serve.

# Baked Eggs

Servings: 4

Preparation time: 10 minutes

Cooking time: 12 minutes

## Ingredients:

- 1 cup of marinara sauce, divided
- 1 tablespoon of capers, drained and divided
- 8 eggs
- ¼ cup of whipping cream, divided
- ¼ cup of low-fat Parmesan cheese, shredded and divided
- Salt and ground black pepper, as required
- 4 cups of fresh baby spinach

## Instructions:

1. Grease 4 ramekins. Set aside.
2. Divide the marinara sauce in the bottom of every prepared ramekin evenly and top with capers.
3. Carefully crack 2 eggs over marinara sauce into each ramekin and top with cream, followed by the Parmesan cheese.

4. Sprinkle each ramekin with salt and black pepper.
5. Select "Bake" of Breville Smart Air Fryer Oven and adjust the temperature to 400 degrees F.
6. Set the timer for 12 minutes and press "Start/Stop" to start preheating.
7. When the unit beeps to point out that it's preheated, arrange the ramekins over the wire rack.
8. When the Cooking time is completed, remove the ramekins from the oven.
9. Serve warm alongside the spinach.

# Spinach & Tomato Bites

Servings: 2

Preparation time: 10 minutes

Cooking time: 30 minutes

## Ingredients:

- 4 eggs
- 1/3 cup of spinach, chopped
- ½ cup of tomatoes, chopped
- ½ cup of unsweetened almond milk
- 1 cup of low-fat Gouda cheese, shredded Salt, as required

## Instructions:

1. In a large ramekin, add all the Ingredients and blend well.
2. Place the ramekins in the air fry basket.
3. Select "Air Fry" of Breville Smart Air Fryer Oven and adjust the temperature to 340 degrees F.
4. Set the timer for 30 minutes and press "Start/Stop" to start preheating.

5. When the unit beeps to point out that it's preheated, insert the air fry basket in the oven.

6. When the Cooking time is completed, remove the air fry basket from the oven.

7. Serve hot.

# Zucchini Omelet

Servings: 2

Preparation time: 15 minutes

Cooking time: 18 minutes

## Ingredients:

- 1 teaspoon of olive oil
- 1 zucchini, julienned
- 4 eggs
- ¼ teaspoon of fresh basil, chopped
- ¼ teaspoon of red pepper flakes, crushed
- Salt and ground black pepper, as required

## Instructions:

1. In a skillet, heat the oil over medium heat and cook the zucchini for about 4-5 minutes.
2. Remove from the heat and put aside to chill slightly.
3. Meanwhile, in a bowl, add the eggs, basil, red pepper flakes, salt and black pepper and beat until well combined.
4. In a baking dish, place the zucchini mixture.

5. Top with egg mixture and gently stir to mix.

6. Select "Air Fry" of Breville Smart Air Fryer Oven and adjust the temperature to 355 degrees F.

7. Set the timer for 10 minutes and press "Start/Stop" to start preheating.

8. When the unit beeps to point out that it's preheated, arrange the baking dish over the wire rack.

9. When the Cooking time is completed, remove the baking dish from oven and transfer the omelette onto a plate.

10. Cut into equal-sized wedges and serve hot.

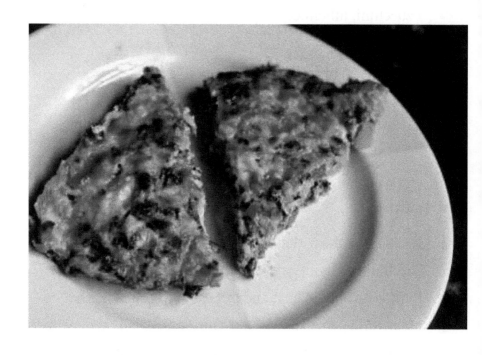

# Bell Pepper Omelet

Servings: 2

Preparation time: 10 minutes

Cooking time: 10 minutes

## Ingredients:

- 1 teaspoon of coconut oil
- 1 small onion, sliced
- ½ of green bell pepper, seeded and chopped
- 4 eggs
- ¼ teaspoon of unsweetened almond milk
- Salt and ground black pepper, as required
- ¼ cup of low-fat Cheddar cheese, grated

## Instructions:

1. In a skillet, melt the coconut oil over medium heat and cook the onion and bell pepper for about 4-5 minutes.
2. Remove the skillet from heat and put aside to chill slightly.
3. Meanwhile, in a bowl, add the eggs, milk, salt and black pepper and beat well.

4. Add the cooked onion mixture and gently stir to mix.

5. Place the bell pepper mixture into a little baking dish.

6. Select "Air Fry" of Breville Smart Air Fryer Oven and adjust the temperature to 355 degrees F.

7. Set the timer for 10 minutes and press "Start/Stop" to start preheating.

8. When the unit beeps to point out that it's preheated, arrange the baking dish over the wire rack.

9. When the Cooking time is completed, remove the baking dish from  oven and place onto a wire rack to chill for about 5 minutes before serving.

10. Cut the omelets into 2 portions and serve hot.

# Bell Pepper & Broccoli Omelet

Servings: 4

Preparation time: 10 minutes

Cooking time: 2 hours

## Ingredients:

- 6 eggs
- ½ cup of unsweetened almond milk
- 1/8 teaspoon of red chili powder
- 1/8 teaspoon of garlic powder
- Salt and ground black pepper, as required
- 1 medium red bell pepper, seeded and sliced thinly
- 1 cup of small broccoli florets
- 1 small yellow onion, chopped
- 2 tablespoons of fresh parsley, chopped

## Instructions:

1. In a bowl, add the eggs, milk, chili powder, garlic powder, salt and black pepper and beat until well combined.
2. In a baking dish, mix the bell pepper, broccoli and onion.
3. Pour the egg mixture on top and gently stir to mix.

4. Arrange the baking dish over the wire rack.

5. Select "Slow Cooker" of Breville Smart Air Fryer Oven and assail "High".

6. Set the timer for 1½-2 hours and press "Start/Stop" to start cooking.

7. When the Cooking time is completed, remove the baking dish from the oven and transfer the omelets onto a serving plate.

8. Cut into 4 equal-sized wedges and serve hot with the garnishing of parsley.

# Mixed Veggie Omelet

Servings: 6

Preparation time: 15 minutes

Cooking time: 2 hours 13 minutes

## Ingredients:

- 1 tablespoon of olive oil
- 1 medium onion, chopped
- ¾ cup of carrot, peeled and chopped
- ¾ cup of zucchini, chopped
- ¼ cup of green bell pepper, seeded and chopped
- ¼ cup of red bell pepper, seeded and chopped
- ½ cup of low-fat Parmesan cheese, grated
- 8 eggs
- Salt and ground black pepper, as required

## Instructions:

1. In a skillet, heat the oil over medium heat and cook the onion for about 2-3 minutes.
2. Add the remaining vegetables and cook for about 8-10 minutes.

3. Remove from the heat and put aside to chill slightly.

4. Meanwhile, in a bowl, add cheese, eggs and black pepper and beat until well combined.

5. In a baking dish, place the vegetable mixture.

6. Pour the egg mixture on top evenly.

7. Arrange the baking dish over the wire rack.

8. Select "Slow Cooker" of Breville Smart Air Fryer Oven and assail "High".

9. Set the timer for two hours and press "Start/Stop" to start cooking.

10. When the Cooking time is completed, remove the baking dish from the oven and transfer the omelets onto a serving plate.

11. Cut into equal-sized wedges and serve hot.

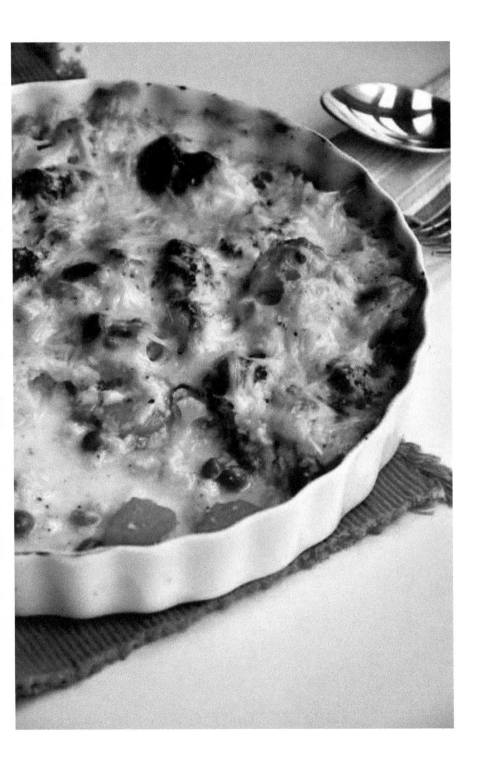

Lightning Source UK Ltd.
Milton Keynes UK
UKHW020729210621
385887UK00005B/166